How to Turn Your

Boyfriend

into a

Love Slave

& other spells

to inspire passion, romance, and seduction

Deborah Gray

illustrated by Sue Ninham

HarperSanFrancisco

A Division of HarperCollins*Publishers*

HarperCollins books may be purchased for educational, business, or sales promotional use. For information please write: Special Markets Department, HarperCollins Publishers, Inc., 10 East 53rd Street, New York, NY 10022.

HarperCollins Web site: http://www.harpercollins.com

HarperCollins®, ♨®, and HarperSanFrancisco™ are trademarks of HarperCollins Publishers, Inc.

FIRST EDITION

Library of Congress Cataloging-in-Publication Data
Gray, Deborah
How to turn your boyfriend into a love slave & other spells to
    inspire passion, romance, and seduction / Deborah Gray; illustrated
    by Sue Ninham.
        p. cm.
ISBN 0–06–251732–5 (pbk.)
1. Witchcraft and sex. 2. Love–Miscellanea. 3. Magic.
4. Goddess religion. I. Title.
BF1572.S4 G73 2000
133.4'42–dc21   00–047277

01 02 03 05 06 QF 10 9 8 7 6 5 4 3 2 1

Contents

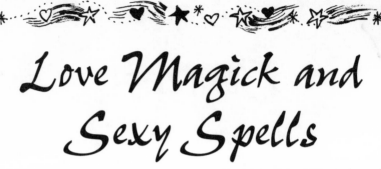

Love Magick and Sexy Spells

Love magick and sexy spells are as ancient and natural as love itself.

The art of seduction has always been synonymous with the art of magick and enchantment. Just take a look at two of the world's most famous Love Goddesses, Aphrodite and Venus – these gorgeous immortals are not only beautiful archetypes of true love, femininity and sexiness, but they're also experts at powerful magick and bewitchery who can whip up a fabulous love spell to win over any intended lover in a goddess minute.

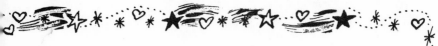

In ancient times, sexy love magick was considered
to be perfectly normal and natural, and no
self-respecting *mortal goddess* would ever go out on a
social occasion without a love spell or a magick
potion tucked alongside her eye kohl and lip rouge
(just in case she came upon a likely candidate
for a passionate and lusty rendezvous).
What fun parties they must have had!

Even nowadays, all you have to do is mention
the magickal art of love and seduction to someone,
and which sexy diva comes into most people's minds?
Why, Queen Cleopatra of course! She was
not only one of the most famous women on the
planet, who helped put the art of seduction into the
history books, but she was also another powerful

enchantress who cleverly cast erotic love
spells and magick potions to seduce whoever took her
fancy. And those love spells sure must have helped,
'cause apparently she was not particularly beautiful.
Yet neither the powerful statesman Julius Caesar,
nor the young and hunky Mark Antony, seemed to mind
being captured by her feminine wiles
and spellbound by her witchy ways.

Of all the millions of divas throughout history,
these more *bewitching* and magickal goddesses are
among the most popular and copied sex symbols of all
time, and seem to be the image many women relate to
in either past life memories or reincarnations!
And why is that? Well, it could be that most of us
can absolutely relate to that compelling desire for the

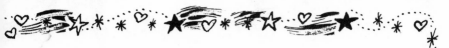

ultimate love experience – and let's face it, we are all born with a natural urge for love and passion.

More than any other aspect of our human existence, our search for eternal love is the most basic and strong desire of all. Love and sex is the natural connection we can all relate to. Since time began, men and women have been stirring up secret love potions, discovering powerful aphrodisiacs and casting magick spells to not only enhance their sexual allure but to help attract and help keep their lover and soul mate faithful and perfectly contented.

As the old saying goes, *'Love makes the world go 'round'* – so here's to love, passion and bewitchery, and to the magickal secrets of sexy sorcery!

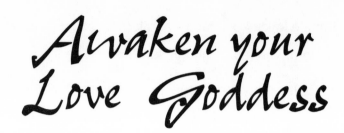

Awaken your Love Goddess

One of the most important steps into bewitchery and spellcasting begins by awakening your own inner magick and mystical power. Each and every aspect of our lives and relationships can be energized and strengthened by the uplifting power of a magick ritual, but did you know that one of the best ways to empower your love life is to connect with your own special Love Goddess?

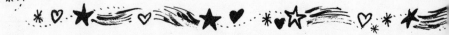

There are many different goddesses from the
various pantheons of ancient magick, and they all
resonate with their own enchanting energy. While
each of them can be called on to
empower any type of ritual you like, your own
special Love Goddess is cosmically aligned with
the vibrations of your deep subconscious – her
sensual energy can help you awaken your own
true magickal nature and seductive power.

To help you find your special Love Goddess,
look up your star sign on the following pages
and see which ancient enchantress can help
you weave your magick spells for passion,
love and seduction.

Aries

The Goddess MAIA personifies your Aries sense
of playfulness and sexy energy. Maia is the
goddess of fertility and fiery passion who was
honored by the ancient Romans with fabulous all-
night toga parties and flower-stomping
festivals. She is the ideal goddess to ensure that
you always exude that special enchanting
glow, whether you've been
up dancing 'til dawn in your bare feet,
or when you're simply relaxing at home with your
chosen one – preferably sipping red wine
in front of a cosy fire.

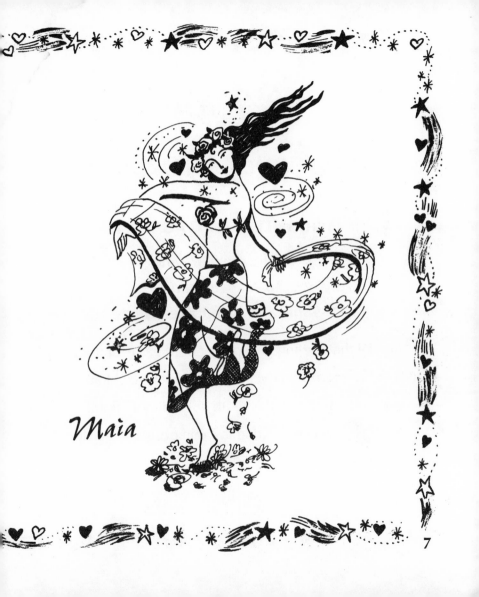

Maia

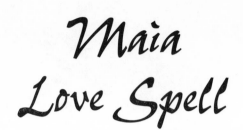

Maia
Love Spell

YOU WILL NEED TO GATHER:

A red scarf or robe
An orange candle
Your favorite floral essence

Invoke the sizzling love power of Maia by draping a red scarf or robe over your shoulders. Light an orange candle anointed with your favorite floral essence, then sit in a comfortable position nearby.

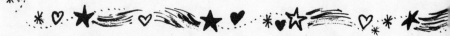

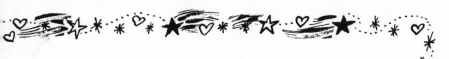

Breathe deeply and concentrate on drawing loving energy towards you. Picture the goddess in your mind as you repeat this incantation:

'Weave your spell of silken thread,
Draped with deepest velvet-red,
Through cedar woods and ancient pine;
Surround me with love and romance divine.

O fairest Maia, goddess of desire,
Through indigo clouds of incense and fire,
Let her earthly guide be candle glow,
Into the temple may passion flow.'

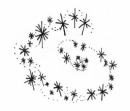

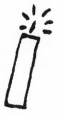

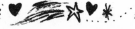

Stay With Me

YOU WILL NEED TO GATHER:

Seven small stones
A cup of tarragon leaves
A box

If you'd like to attract a great guy (or girl) and
you want this new love to last, help cement the
relationship by casting this spell on the night of
a new moon. Gather together seven small stones (they
may be pebbles from a garden or crystals bought from
a shop) and a cup of tarragon leaves.

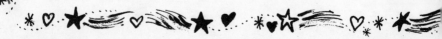

Go to a quiet space in your home near a window.
Place the stones clockwise in a circle around you
while you think about your intended lover. Sprinkle
the tarragon around in an anti-clockwise direction as
you repeat this incantation:

'Solid to the right, strength is on the left,
Our love will stay with the power of this
The Magick Hour.'

Finish the spell by remaining within the circle for
a few minutes while you concentrate on visualizing
the two of you happy and in love. Leave the circle as
it is overnight. In the morning, gather up the stones
and tarragon and put them in a box to keep under
your bed.

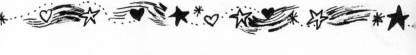

Taurus

Your goddess was worshipped in ancient Crete. Represented by the female bull, her name is TAUROPOLOS. Honored for her strength and the ability to bring out lust in everyone, young men would line up, eagerly showing off their physical prowess by attempting somersaults through her magnificent horns. A warning though: her powers of attraction could be dangerously irresistible, so do be careful when you wear that sexy red underwear, or you may find yourself being chased around a field by a Latin gymnast!

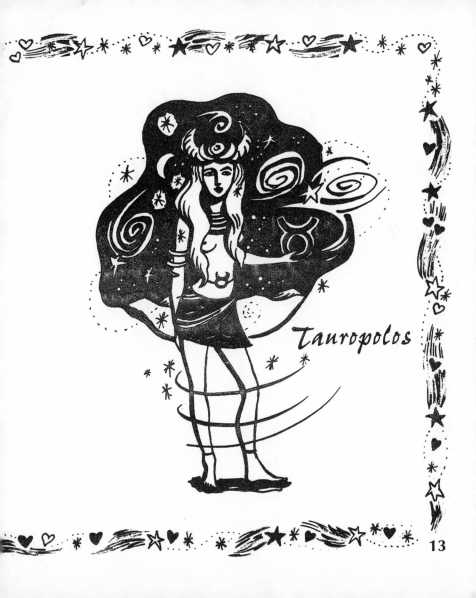

Tauropolos

Tauropolos Love Spell

Ask the Goddess Tauropolos to help bring love into your life by casting this spell on the night of a new or growing moon. Gather together some saffron powder, a pebble (one that you have found outside in a park or a garden) and a garnet crystal (available from crystal shops or new age stores).

Take a bath or shower to clear away any negative or stressful energy and put on some clean, natural-fiber clothing. Find a quiet, private space in your home and place the pebble and crystal on the floor in front of you. Sprinkle the saffron around you in a clockwise

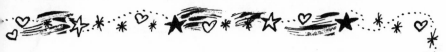

circle as you concentrate on feeling the goddess
energy. Repeat this incantation:

> *'See here now the saffron dust*
> *Swirling at your feet,*
> *Turning now to fiery jewels*
> *And precious magick gems.*
> *I look again – your secret name*
> *Is carved in whitest stone.*
> *I call on you Tauropolos, goddess of ancient Crete,*
> *May romance knock upon my door*
> *and love's delight be shown.'*

Seal the spell's power by sweeping up the saffron with
a broom. Place the items of enchantment in a wooden
or cardboard box and keep it in your bedroom for at
least a month.

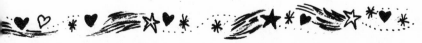

Heart's Desire

When you are ready for someone new or to bring back a past love, cast this attraction spell on a fine morning of a new or waxing moon (when the moon is growing from new to full).

Begin by finding a safe place outside your home where you can see the front door or a front window. Take a handful of sesame seeds with you and stand for a few moments looking into the sky as you appreciate the different shades of blue and the different shapes and colors of any clouds above you. Fill your lungs

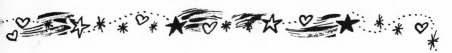

with fresh air by taking a number of deep breaths.
Then sprinkle the sesame seeds near the front door
and window of your home, repeating this incantation:

> *'My heart's desire will now fully bloom,*
> *My true soul mate will be arriving soon.*
> *As the seeds of magick begin to grow,*
> *Through my door real love shall flow.'*

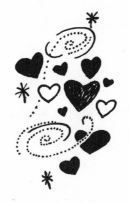

Gemini

NIKE, goddess of expression and movement, is your perfect twin. She is a beautiful winged nymph who zooms through the skies at great speed and loves hanging out with her groovy goddess friends. Nike always makes sure she's invited to the best A-list parties in heaven. (Remember this whenever a snooty doorman is giving you problems!) Most importantly, Nike is the goddess of victory who always gets her man. Her energy aligns perfectly with your incredible zest for life and love of good company.

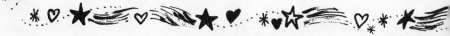

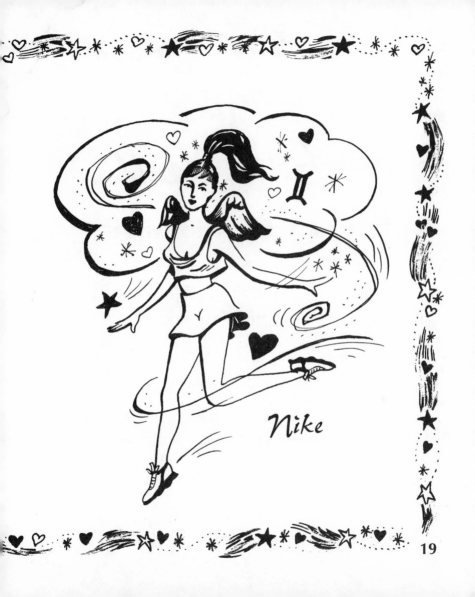

Nike

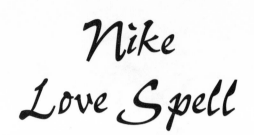

Nike Love Spell

YOU WILL NEED TO GATHER:

A silver ring or necklace
A white feather
A sprig of lavender

To invoke love and the power of Nike, gather together your items of enchantment. At night, put on the necklace or ring and hold the feather and lavender in your hands. Stand near an open

window in your home, look into the sky and whisper
this incantation to the night wind:

> *'Since time began to soar and fly,*
> *It is written on the wind:*
> *Fairest Nike shall bring success*
> *Sent on a goddess wing.*
> *Here this night I call on you*
> *To ensure love's destiny,*
> *May your enchantment light my way*
> *And bring eternal joy to me.'*

Seal the spell's power by breathing in the aroma of
the lavender for a moment and then tossing both the
feather and lavender out of the window.

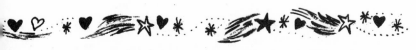

Bliss Bath

YOU WILL NEED TO GATHER:

1 cup Epsom salts
½ cup baking soda
1 tablespoon dried lavender
1 teaspoon chamomile tea

Treat your own mind and body to some love magick with this wonderful bath of bliss. Begin by mixing up some 'bliss powder,' using the ingredients above.

Mix together the ingredients in a large bowl and let them stand for one hour. If you wish, you can

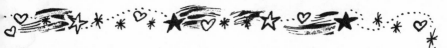

also add a few drops of your or favorite essential oil. Then put everything into a jar with a lid. Draw a warm bath and pour in a few tablespoons of the 'bliss powder.' Soak in the bath while you relax your body and mind completely.

Cancer

SELENE is the ancient Roman goddess of the moon and emotional love. Her skin glimmers like silver – legend has it that she carefully bathes in the sea at sunset before traveling across the night sky in a glistening chariot to woo her admirers with wondrous poetry and romance. With your love of expensive perfumes and candlelit baths, Selene is the perfect goddess for you to call upon before you invite your lover over for a seductive night of moonlit passion.

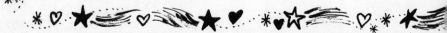

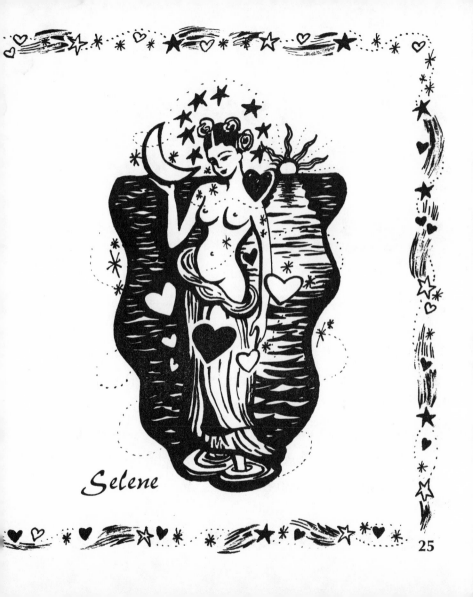

Selene

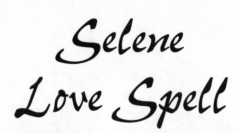

Selene Love Spell

Empower yourself with the energy of the Goddess Selene with this ancient bathing ritual. Perform this ritual on a night before a hot date, or whenever you feel like boosting your powers of attraction.

Take some time out to pamper yourself with a lovely bubble bath or fragrant shower. Remain in the shower or bath for a few moments as you imagine that Selene's energy is shining through to you and filling you with her enchanted power. Then, after you dry yourself, anoint your body with a lightly perfumed body cream as you repeat this incantation:

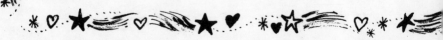

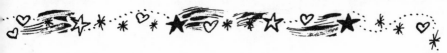

'Sylphs and elves gather to see,
That Goddess Selene shall hearken to me.
Hear my plea in night's quietest hour,
Let your moonlight glisten with silvery power.
May each dusk and dawn
Bring me love's true glimmer,
For it shall be so and so will it be.'

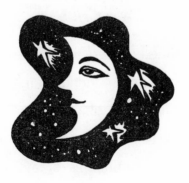

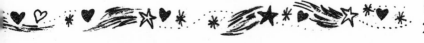

Chocolate Heart Spell

YOU WILL NEED TO GATHER:

A heart-shaped box of chocolates
Lavender cologne
A red ribbon

Spice up the time-honored gift of a beautiful box of chocolates with some seduction sorcery. Before you give it to your intended, place the box of chocolates on a small table, then walk clockwise once around it as you lightly spray a fine mist of lavender cologne in

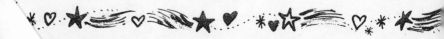

the air. Next, stand near the table and face east.
Breathe calmly for a few minutes and repeat this
incantation:

> *'Spirit of the eastern sun*
> *Now my charming has begun,*
> *All true beauty that lies within,*
> *Seal this spell with love to win.*
> *In the name of good it will be done.'*

Finish the spell by tying a red ribbon around the
box of chocolates.

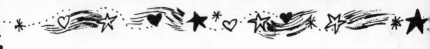

Leo

Just like you, BAST is the original sex kitten.
This Egyptian goddess understands the joy of
the hunt, and she aligns perfectly with your sexy
feline psyche. It is said that just one look
from her golden almond eyes can entice
anyone she chooses.

A favorite goddess among the women of
Nefertiti's time, Bast is an ancient solar deity
who also takes the form of a cat or lion.
She particularly enjoys playfully toying with
her lovers before she finally captures them.
(Sound familiar?)

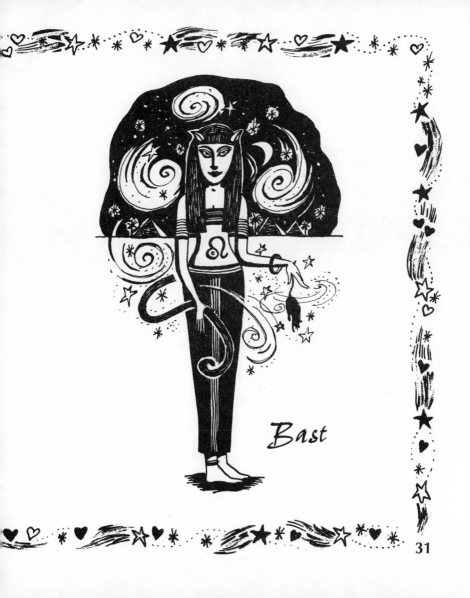

Bast

Bast Love Spell

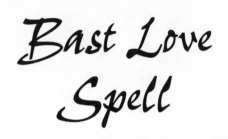

YOU WILL NEED TO GATHER:

A stick of musk incense
A leopard-print or tiger-print scarf
A tiger's eye crystal

To help bring romance and the energy of the Goddess
Bast into your love life, gather together
your items of enchantment. At 7 o'clock on any night,
light the incense and wrap the animal-print scarf
around you. Hold the crystal in both hands
and breathe deeply and calmly for a few moments.

Concentrate on attracting love toward you and picture the goddess in your mind as you say these magick words:

'O goddess, I see you gaze through golden eyes;
So silently you speak your words.
A delicate stroll through crystal sands,
Curling through perfumed corridors,
Now let this ancient alchemy awaken you O Bast,
Let my desire for sacred love come to me at last.'

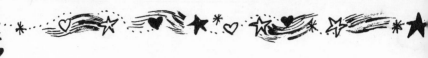

Honeymoon Magick

To bless a new relationship, invite your lover over for supper. A few hours beforehand, purchase or make your own apple cake mix. Blend the ingredients together in a big china bowl and pour the mixture into a baking tin. Sprinkle in a touch of cinnamon and a teaspoon of honey as you repeat this incantation:

'This blessed moon cake that I bake,
Fill up with goodness for everlasting sake.'

After the cake has finished baking, allow it to cool and then hold it up towards the moonlight as you think about your new love and repeat the incantation three more times. When you serve the cake to your lover, don't cut it with a knife or any other cutting tool (this will cut the spell's power). Instead, break off small pieces with your hands and romantically feed the cake to him and then to yourself. Serve with lashings of honey or apple butter for a night of sweet love.

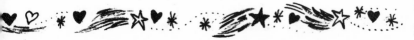

Virgo

Often thought of as an earthy forest nymph, you are also influenced by the star goddess, ASTRAEA. She became bored with earthly pursuits and rose elegantly into the sky to form the constellation of Virgo. Astraea believes in fair play and loyalty, but no man should ever underestimate her gentle nature, or she will be gone in a shimmering flash of stardust. Just like you, she can just as easily enjoy flying away on her own (preferably first-class) to somewhere exotic and fabulous if she needs some extra stimulation and excitement.

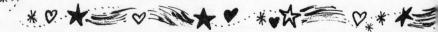

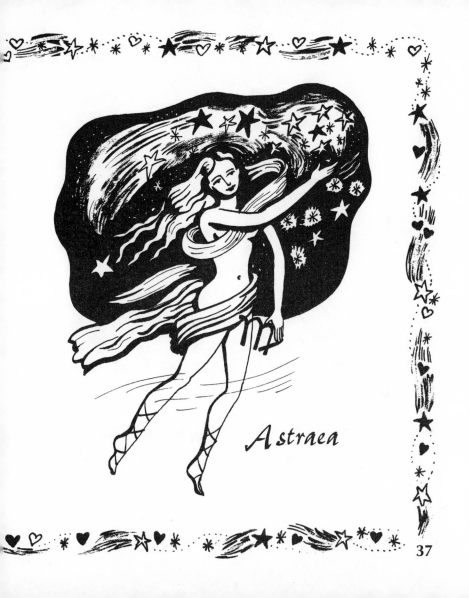

Astraea

Astraea Love Spell

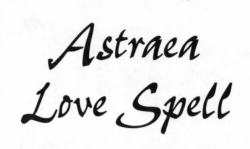

YOU WILL NEED TO GATHER:

A peridot or green crystal

Geranium-scented body oil

A small make-up mirror

Tissue paper

A pretty gift box

A piece of blue paper

All goddesses adore beautiful presents, so attract love and Astraea into your home by making her a special magick box. Gather together a peridot or a

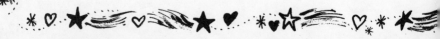

green crystal (available at new age and crystal shops), a small vial of geranium-scented body oil, and a small make-up mirror. Wrap everything in tissue and put it into a pretty gift box. Sit down and write these words on a piece of blue paper:

> *'O Goddess Astraea, send me the gift of love*
> *And linger here awhile,*
> *For behold within this magick box*
> *You'll find enchanted fare.*
> *A crystal to shine and light your day*
> *With a secret oil to smooth your care*
> *And a looking glass to guide your way.'*

Put the paper in the box, put on the lid and leave it near your bedroom window for as long as you wish.

Que Sera Sera

YOU WILL NEED TO GATHER:

Two pink candles
Essence of jasmine
Two candle holders
A new notebook

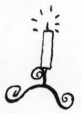

When you want to attract your perfect match, this spell works very well if you concentrate not just on physical appearance, but also on personality and character.

Cast your love spell on the night of a full moon by anointing two pink candles with some essence of jasmine and placing them in holders on either side of a new notebook. Light the candles and sit nearby so you can write down these magick words:

'I call on one who is happy and wise,
Who looks at me with sparkling eyes.
And in his sight I can do no wrong,
For our love is right and true and strong.
So shall the Universe hear my request.'

When you have finished writing, look at the words and, in your mind's eye, concentrate on seeing your new lover; try to feel yourself holding him and send him your affection and thoughts. Repeat the spell once a week for at least a month.

Libra

HATHOR, the Egyptian goddess of art, femininity and beauty, is a wonderful flirt who enjoys lilting music and playing to an audience. So, when you next feel the urge to dance on top of the restaurant table, you'll know it's because your guardian goddess often cheered up the moody gods with an impromptu belly dance around the heavens. Hathor's powers of seduction are among the strongest of all the goddesses, so she's very handy to call on to give you a sexy boost after a hard day of balancing your life (and everyone else's!).

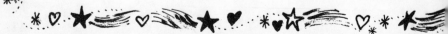

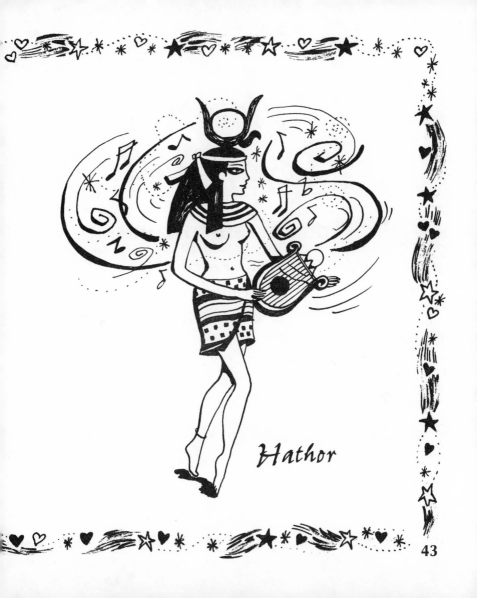

Hathor

Hathor Love Spell

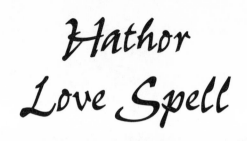

YOU WILL NEED TO GATHER:

Flower petals
Glitter
Morris bells

Attract love and celebrate your connection with the Goddess Hathor by having a little private dance party in her honor. Sprinkle lots of pretty flower petals and glitter over the floor and tie some traditional Morris bells around your wrists and ankles for extra magick

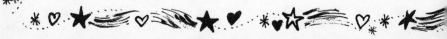

during your goddess dance. You can make Morris bells
by threading a few small craft bells onto some lengths
of pink or red ribbon, and tying them around your
ankles with a bow. (Craft bells are available in
haberdasheries and pet shops.)

Put on some of your favorite music and dance
around your bedroom or living room as you
say aloud:

'O beautiful Hathor, goddess of love,
Send me romance and luck from above.
Let ancient drums beat and ringing bells sound,
Come dance with me as the finest ribbons fly.
Gently walk among Earth's scented flowers,
Shower me from the heavens with love's
sacred power.'

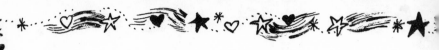

Cupid's Dart

What better way of meeting someone new than holding a party for a number of your friends – making sure, of course, that they invite some of their other friends. This will give you the perfect opportunity to place symbols of togetherness and love discreetly around the rooms to stimulate romantic interest and lots of fun.

The best time to throw the party would be on a Friday evening. Prepare beforehand some plates of passion power food such as fresh fruit and handfuls

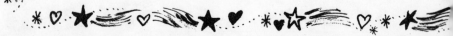

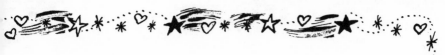

of chocolates and nuts. Place these around your
home for romantic nibbles. You may set a table with
a white tablecloth and make a lovely display of red
and white scented flowers. Then, just before your
guests arrive, walk clockwise around the main room
and say:

'Goddess Venus call Eros here tonight,
If love can start may Cupid's dart find its path.'

Scorpio

The mysterious SERKET is one of the most ancient Egyptian goddesses, who also aligns beautifully with your deep understanding of mysticism and karma. She loves exploring secret and out-of-the-way places and playing sexy mind games with her chosen lovers. You will definitely relate to her way-out dress sense – she loves to wear a stunning scorpion-shaped headdress – and to her passionate sense of her own seductive spiritual power.

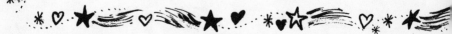

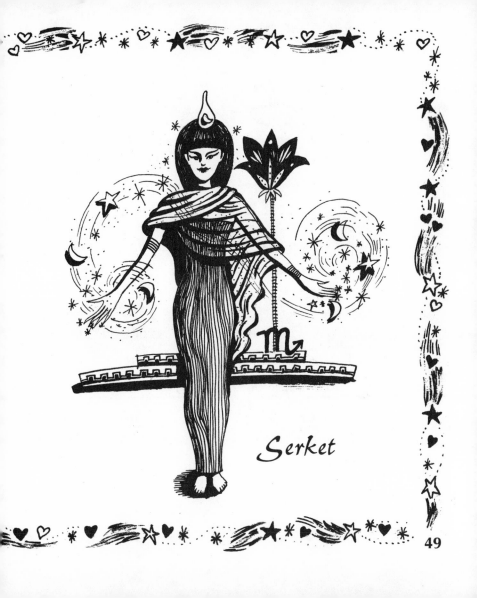

Serket

Serket
Love Spell

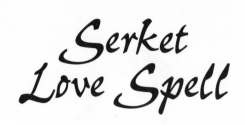

YOU WILL NEED TO GATHER:

A small white party candle
A small purple party candle
Musk oil

To invoke love and your inner goddess power, gather
two small party candles – a white one to represent
yourself and a purple one for Serket. Place the
candles in holders or on a dish, in the center of a
table. Dab a little musk oil onto both candles. Next,
light them both and repeat this incantation:

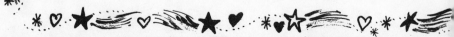

*'I light the flame of mystery
For you, O Goddess Serket,
To unlock the secret pathways
through the magick of ancient Egypt.
As you follow the flickering golden light
Of this enchanted fire,
May you surround me now
With the wonders of love and
passion's true desire.'*

Gaze at the lit candles while you let go of stress and negative thoughts. Watch the candles burn down until the flame goes out and just the wax remains. Leave the melted wax to cool overnight. In the morning, bury it in a garden or flowerpot.

Totally Devoted

the ("Love Slave" spell)

YOU WILL NEED TO GATHER:

Two lengths of string, about 12 inches long
A stick of geranium or ylang ylang incense
Something your intended lover
has touched (eg a pen or a sheet of paper)
A handful of rose petal potpourri

If you want to bring a loved one closer to you,
collect together these items of enchantment on
Friday, the day of Venus. Wrap one of the lengths

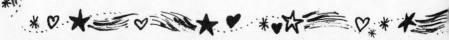

of string around the stick of incense at the base and keep wrapping all the way up to the tip as you focus your mind on your intended and say:

> *'I bind this chord to show my love,*
> *I bind this chord to start desire.'*

Put the item your loved one has touched next to the incense and start wrapping that up with the other piece of string. After you have wrapped everything up, sprinkle the rose petals over the top. For added passion, keep everything under your bed for at least a month.

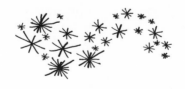

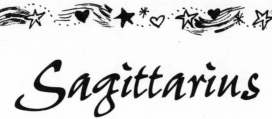

Sagittarius

If you can picture yourself dressed in gold on a dazzling white steed, your hair flying in the wind, then the equine goddess of ancient Gaul, EPONA, is the girl for you. She is fiercely independent, but never knocks back a chance to race some of the fastest men in the west to the finish line. Just like you, Epona is full of surprises and when she does decide to give a guy a break and let him catch her, she lets down her flowing mane and entertains her rapt audience with amazing imitations of lusty bird songs.

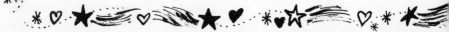

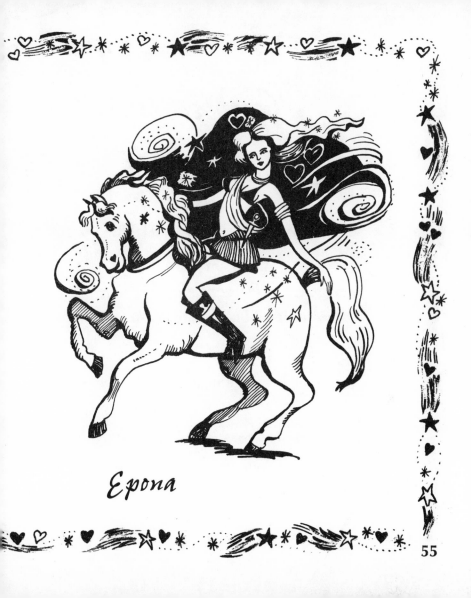

Epona

Epona Love Spell

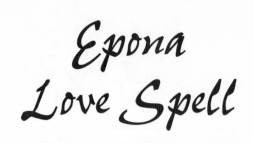

YOU WILL NEED TO GATHER:

Aloe vera gel
A leather belt
A natural-bristle hairbrush

To invoke the love power of the Goddess Epona, collect your spell items during the week of a waxing (growing) moon. At 8 o'clock on any evening, take a luxurious bath or shower. After you have patted yourself dry, anoint your whole body with the aloe

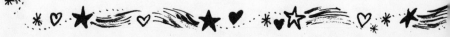

as you concentrate your mind on thoughts of love and romance. Remain undressed and wrap the leather belt around your waist. Gently brush your hair as you look into a mirror and repeat this magick incantation:

'Hearken now and ride alongside the unicorn,
Let's stop to drink at love's sweet well.
Lie among Apollo's garden of meadow fern;
I call you here O wild Epona.
Come show me again the highest magick realm,
This enchanted land where passion is born.'

After your ritual, keep the belt and the brush in a special corner of your bedroom.

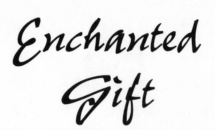

Enchanted Gift

What better symbol of love than a beautiful handmade gift. This lucky talisman is easy to make and it's a wonderful magick charm for a lover or friend.

Make a little pouch of satin or cotton, in your loved one's favorite color. Then find a nicely shaped light-colored pebble or small stone and a blue indelible marker pen. Wash and dry the stone, then hold it to your 'third eye chakra' – between your eyes – as you visualize a golden light shining from your chakra, and flowing into the stone.

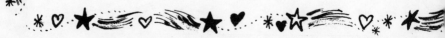

Think of things your loved one desires and needs most in their life. Choose one and, as you concentrate strongly on that, repeat this incantation:

'May this stone help their dream come true,
With loving and generous energy,
By the ancient rule of three times three,
May this now be done so mote it be.'

Finally, draw the number '7' onto the stone. Place it into the pouch for an inspiring magickal gift from your heart.

Capricorn

The Roman nymph ALMATHEIA once nourished
Zeus, king of the gods, with goat's milk and honey.
A cheeky and ambitious goddess, she was
rewarded with the gift of everlasting success and
tenacity and the ability to sustain the world.
Almatheia's feisty energy fits right in with your
Capricornian talent for whipping up a
post-l'amour meal out of the one egg and leftover
champagne in your fridge. (Although your lover
probably needs a bit more nourishing than that
to keep up with your incredible stamina!)

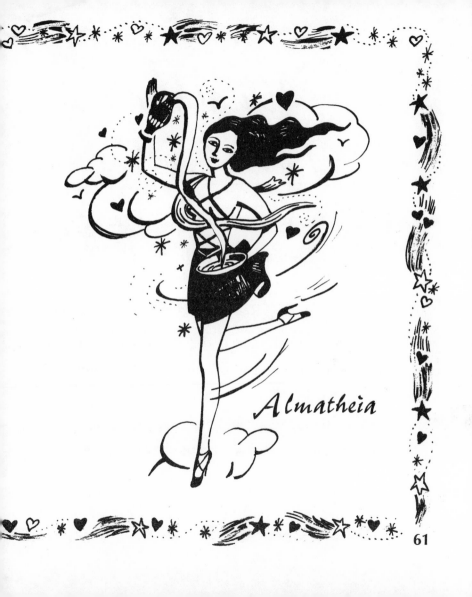

Almatheia

Almatheia Love Spell

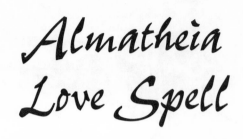

YOU WILL NEED TO GATHER:

Jasmine-scented body oil
A small sprig of fresh mint, finely chopped
A cup of goat's milk

To bring love and the power of Almatheia toward you, cast this spell on the day of Saturn, Saturday. Find a time in the day or evening when you can be undisturbed for a while and place all your spell items in your bathroom. Take a relaxing shower or, better

still, a bath. While you are bathing, smooth some of the body oil over yourself while you think of your love wish. After bathing, dry yourself and pour the goat's milk into a cup. Sprinkle the mint into the goat's milk. Take a sip, then repeat this incantation:

'Let me bathe with you, O sacred one
In the nectar of the gods.
Let the coolest mint soothe your brow
As you sip the milk of love.
Let scented oils bring you near
O Goddess Almatheia;
Send me the elixir of romance and laughter
And a joyous dream so dear.'

Finish the spell by drinking the goat's milk and the mint. Repeat the incantation as often as you like.

Bubble Bubble

YOU WILL NEED TO GATHER:

A cauldron or metal bowl
Two silver candles
One maroon candle
Jasmine incense
A wooden stick

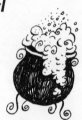

You've seen the guy you want, you just have to get his attention! Leave your magick cauldron or metal bowl near a window to be charged by the moon overnight.

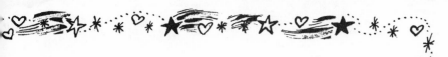

On the next night, place the bowl on a table between
two silver candles. Place a maroon candle in the bowl
by melting the end of the candle slightly with a match
so it sticks firmly to the bottom of the bowl. Light the
incense and the silver candles. With the wooden stick
in your right hand, gently tap the side of the bowl
three times as you say the words:

> *'One to reach him, two to bring him,*
> *Three to keep him near.'*

Tap the cauldron with the stick three more times. Light
the maroon candle as you picture your intended lover
in your mind, focusing on loving thoughts. Seal the
spell's power by snuffing out the candles and saying:

> *'Devoted we'll be, together as one,*
> *It shall be so, this spell is done'.*

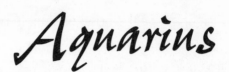

Aquarius

You are aligned with the Egyptian sky goddess, NUUT, the personification of heavenly love power. Her sensuous body is painted with stars and she is able to reach out with her delicate fingers and toes to touch the four cardinal points of the world. (No wonder you can so easily stretch your credit-card limit to the north, south, east and west!) Her spiritual energy fits perfectly with the inventive way you can think of three lovers at once and your eerie ability to attract interesting lovers from faraway places.

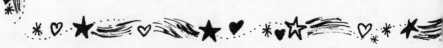

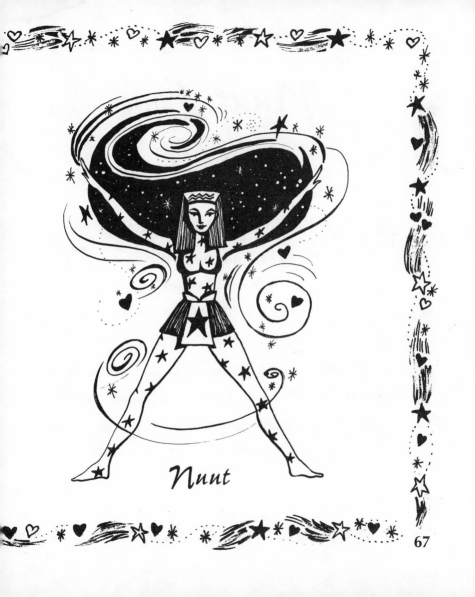

Nuut

Nuut Love Spell

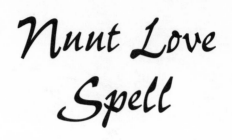

YOU WILL NEED TO GATHER:

Three floating silver candles
A bowl of water
Rose incense
Sugar

To call in romance and the power of the Goddess Nuut, you could try a little love magick by casting this spell on a Friday, preferably during a new or waxing (growing) moon. Place three floating silver candles in a

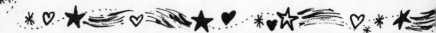

bowl of water. Light the candles and one stick of rose incense. Sit nearby as you focus your thoughts on romance and love, while gently inhaling the aroma of the incense. Next, sprinkle a tiny amount of sugar into the bowl of water as you repeat this incantation:

'I stir, I mix, I manifest the energy of Goddess Nuut.
These words I speak, this magick spell
Her power will invoke.
I stir, I mix, I manifest the casting has begun;
A thousand stars adorn her O the Ancient One;
May joy now fill my waking hours
And all my sleep-filled nights.
Send me all my heart's desire
And love that's true and right.'

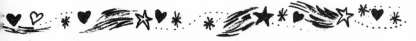

Matchmaker

To encourage your intended lover to think of you, either find a photograph of him or write his name on a clean piece of paper twelve times. Stick it face-down on a small make-up mirror. Then write the following words on the back of a photograph of yourself:

'By these magick words I make this plea,
When you see your reflection
You will think of me.'

Stick the photo on the back of the mirror face-down. Hold the mirror in your hand and concentrate with all your might on visualizing your intended's face. Repeat the same incantation aloud three times.

Keep the mirror in your purse or pocket for at least a month.

Pisces

ISIS is the Egyptian Goddess of High Magick. Her
dreamy soul and psychic powers match perfectly
with your Piscean spiritual awareness, but, like you,
she can also be the ultimate love diva. Her
powers are legendary – she was one of the first girls
to use glamour and magick spells to entice her
lovers. Her apprentice was the naughty Cleopatra,
who seduced Mark Antony and Julius Caesar with a
lot of help from the magick of Isis. So, if you can get
this goddess on your team, your dreams of running
off with your perfect lover are not too far off.

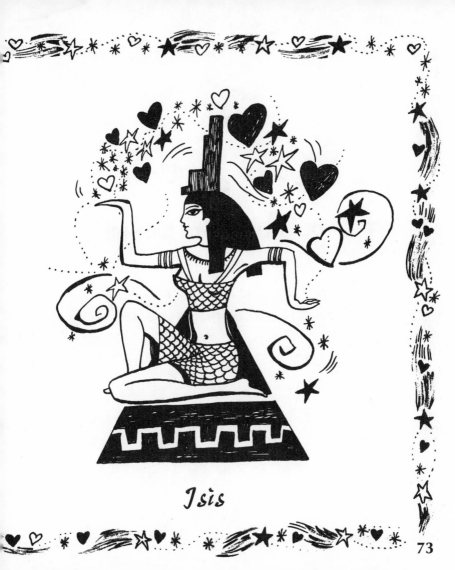

Isis

Isis
Love Spell

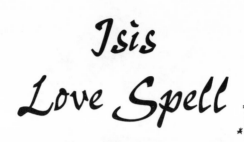

YOU WILL NEED TO GATHER:

A few strands of your own hair
Three camellia or carnation petals
A small amethyst crystal

Use the power of your dreams to bring love and the Goddess Isis into your magick realm. Take a few strands of your own hair (a few from your comb or brush will do fine), plus the camellia or carnation petals and amethyst crystal. Set up a special altar to

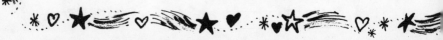

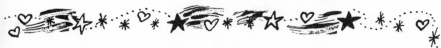

Isis in your bedroom by placing your spell items on a pretty table. Hold the amethyst in your hand and focus on feelings of love and happiness as you repeat this incantation:

'Goddess Isis, lady of the ancient way,
Carry my message through the call of the spirit
Along the sacred river Nile.
Hear me whisper in your dreams
Among the rustling reeds of long-forgotten times.
Hasten now and awaken me to precious love
Throughout the night and day.'

Place the petals, hair and crystal under your pillow and repeat this spell as often as you wish.

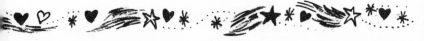

Siren's Song

YOU WILL NEED TO GATHER:

A medium length each of green, mauve and blue wool
Floral perfume

A perfect soul mate is possible for everyone, but for love magick to work effectively, you first need to love and believe completely in yourself. Reflect on that for a while, and then cast this spell at 7 o'clock on a Sunday evening. Gather together the three lengths of

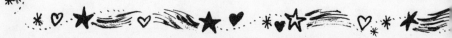

wool and tie them end to end so they form one long strand. Spray a light mist of floral perfume around you and then loosely wrap the strand of wool around your waist. Look at your reflection in a mirror as you say:

> *'From the song of the sirens,*
> *With the call of the mermaid,*
> *I now open myself to receive true love*
> *And never will it fade.'*

Finish by rolling the strand of wool up in a ball and keeping it in a drawer near your bed.

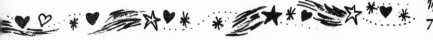

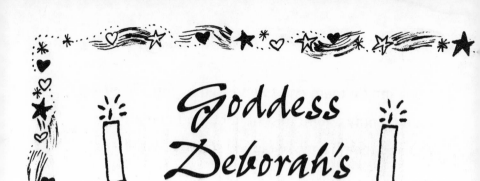

Goddess Deborah's

Favorite Potions and Enchanted Notions

One of my greatest joys is to rummage through my precious collection of ancient recipes and secret potions to find new and exciting ways of weaving a little love magick.

On the following pages are some of my favorite charms, potions and enchanted notions to help you find romance, bring back a past love or meet your perfect match.

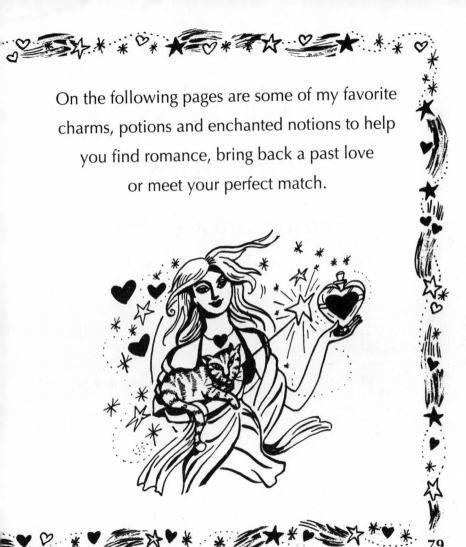

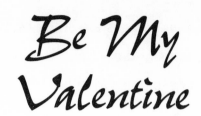

Be My Valentine

YOU WILL NEED TO GATHER:

3 pieces of parchment or recycled paper
A green pencil
A small snip of your own hair

Whether searching for a soul mate, looking for a lost love, or happily married, we could all do with a bit of passion power. What better time to weave a little magick than Valentine's Day! In the days of ancient Rome, February 14th was celebrated as a holiday festival for romance and engagement. The wife

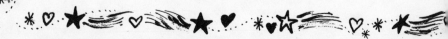

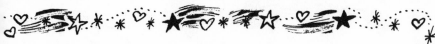

of Jupiter, the Goddess Juno, would bestow her blessings on courting couples to bring good luck and on singles hunting for their ideal lovemate.

Ask Juno for some modern wizardry by casting this spell on the night before Valentine's Day. Use the green pencil to write down the name of your intended lover on each piece of paper, then sprinkle a little of your hair on top of each page. Roll the pieces up one by one, and hold them near your chest. Concentrate on attracting your lover toward you as you say these words:

> *'With goddess power so divine,*
> *I curl my locks as you do mine,*
> *One before and two behind,*
> *Be my only Valentine.'*

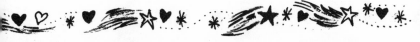

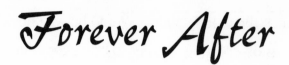

Forever After

YOU WILL NEED TO GATHER:

*A teaspoon each of cinnamon,
marjoram, ginseng, sage and basil
A wooden bowl
A sieve*

Every person you meet and every relationship you
have is a lesson for your soul. Before you are ready
to meet someone new, it is important to clear away
any bitterness over a past relationship, especially if
you have just been through a break-up or you have
regrets. Throw your old worries to the wind with this
great renewal ceremony.

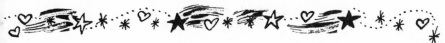

At some time before the ceremony, mix and grind the herbs and spices together in a wooden bowl as you let go of negativity or any bitterness about the old relationship. Next, pour the mixture into a sieve. Discard all but the finest powder. Stand near an open window or go outside to a safe place and throw the magick mixture up in the air, while repeating this incantation:

> *'Here to the sacred wind*
> *Fly my worries and my past,*
> *Out with the old and in with the new,*
> *My true path is clear at last.'*

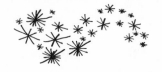

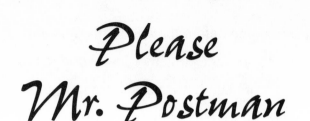

Please Mr. Postman

YOU WILL NEED TO GATHER:

A pink candle
A white candle
A medium-sized pink envelope
Light floral perfume

If your lover is out of town and you'd like to perk up his interest, cast this spell on the night of either a new or a full moon. Sit down at your writing table to write a letter and light one pink and one white candle. Meditate for a few minutes while you think

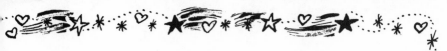

about the one you love. Imagine you are next to him, feeling very contented and happy. As you write your letter, open your mind and heart to let that happiness flow through you. Be spontaneous with what you say to him in the letter.

When you finish writing, spray the folded letter with a light floral perfume and put it into a medium-sized pink envelope. Hold it to your chest as you say:

> *'On this magick night*
> *Fly quickly my words and thoughts*
> *To reach the man I love.'*

Post the letter the next morning at 9 o'clock.

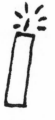

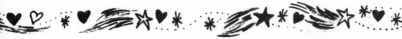

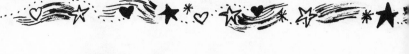

Baby Come Back

YOU WILL NEED TO GATHER:

A small taper candle
A thorn from a pink or red rose
Clove oil
A small red or purple silk drawstring bag

To help bring back an ex-lover, inscribe his initials
with the thorn of a pink or red rose in the side of a
small taper candle. (Use a candle that will burn down
in fifteen or twenty minutes.) Then anoint the candle

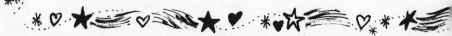

with a drop or two of oil of clove. As you light the candle, visualize your ex-lover's face and repeat this incantation:

> *'This candle is my burning love for you*
> *As bright as the sacred sun.*
> *May this flame warm your spirit*
> *And let us soon be one.'*

Sit back in a comfortable position and gaze at the candle until it melts down into a puddle of wax. Allow the candle flame to go out naturally. When the wax has cooled right down and hardened, put it into the silk bag and tie up the drawstring. For extra attraction power, you can tie the bag to a pretty ribbon and wear it around your neck or place it near the phone for an hour or so each evening.

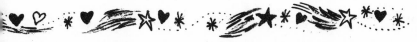

Perfect Reflection

If you are wondering what Mr. or Ms. Right will look like, cast a soul mate reflection spell by gathering a red candle in the evening on a Friday, the day of Venus. Go to a room in which you can see your reflection in a darkened window, light the candle and turn off all electric light.

Gaze at your own eyes and ask any question about your soul mate, such as, 'What will he look like?' Then close your eyes and turn away from the

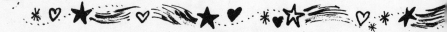

window. After a few seconds, open your eyes and quickly look over your shoulder – you may see their reflection appearing in the window along with yours.

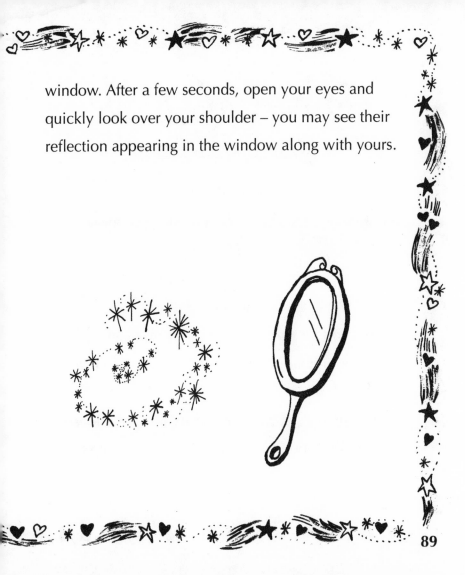

Food of Love

Edible Aphrodisiacs

LICORICE

This aromatic sweet is a very ancient aphrodisiac.

SAGE

This popular kitchen herb is often used in bath oils.

TRUFFLES

The best kind is from a wild mushroom-like fungus that grows in Europe. Expensive but very effective.

EGGS

Apparently many European gypsies feed their lovers a mixture of whipped raw eggs and sugar to keep up sexual stamina.

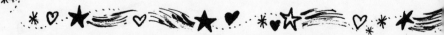

TIRAMISU

Not only does this famous Italian dessert taste divine, it is said to be a powerful aphrodisiac.

FO-TI-TIENG

An ancient Chinese herb that can be sipped in tea before lovemaking.

MUSHROOMS

Lightly cook mushrooms or serve them raw in a salad to arouse the passion within.

OYSTERS

Oysters are a sensuous and exotic addition to any romantic meal.

GINSENG

A well-known herb for stamina and sexuality. Can be taken as a tea or in a vitamin pill.

Tropical
Delight

One of the most ancient and effective aphrodisiacs is
the Polynesian kava root. Polynesian islanders
use kava in important celebrations and love rituals;
they either just nibble on the root or blend powdered
kava with coconut milk.

  The simplest way to make your own exotic
love drink is to mix the following ingredients
in a blender.

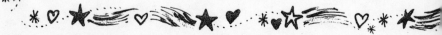

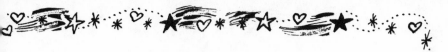

2 teaspoons powdered kava*
1 tablespoon coconut granules or
½ cup coconut milk
½ cup spring water
½ cup soy milk

* If you can't find any kava root, you can use
sweetened cocoa powder as an excellent substitute.

Blend on high for one minute and you'll have enough
for 2 people.

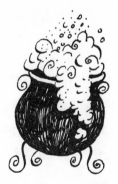

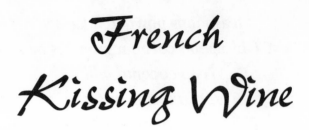

French Kissing Wine

As we all know, the French are renowned for their prowess in both the kitchen and the bedroom. It is said that Josephine used this magick recipe to enchant her Emperor Napoleon. To make French Kissing Wine, mix together the following ingredients in a large bowl.

2 bottles Chablis or light red wine
1 vanilla stick, chopped
a pinch ground cinnamon
1 rhubarb stick, chopped

Let the wine chill in the fridge for 2–3 hours and stir well as you say these words:

> *'Golden sun shine light divine,*
> *Fill with love this wondrous wine.'*

Strain the mixture through a clean cheesecloth and discard the solids. Pour the remaining liquid into a crystal or glass wine decanter to serve with lunch or dinner.

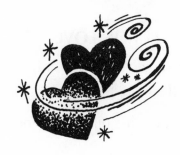

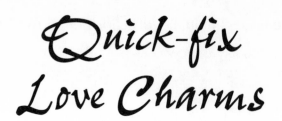

Quick-fix Love Charms

PUMPKIN PASSION

To make an ancient love charm, put seven pumpkin seeds into a small bag of yellow or white cotton. Tie the bag with a gold ribbon and carry it in your pocket or purse.

LEMON LOVE

Cut a heart-shaped piece of peel from a lemon. Place it on a windowsill and let it dry in the sun for seven days. Then wrap it up in a pink cloth and place it under your bed.

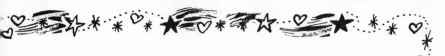

WISHBONE CHARM

To make a love wish come true, save the wishbone from a Christmas turkey and nail it onto your front door on New Year's Day.

TULIP TEASER

To help invite love into your house, keep tulip bulbs in a wooden box somewhere near your front door.

Rose Power
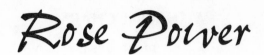

Why wait for that special someone to send you flowers, when you can weave your own spell with the Magick Rose of Love!

I have personally charged the rose on this page with a powerful enchantment. Touch the picture with your right hand, then visualize cuddling your loved one as you repeat these magick words:

'Roses are red,
Violets are blue
The touch of Venus
Shall bring me to you.'

For added power, place a photo of yourself or
your loved one on top of the rose, close this book and
leave it in your bedroom drawer for at least one night.

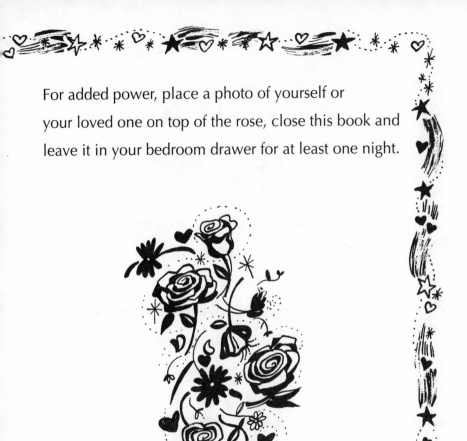

Colors
of Love

Every day of the week has its corresponding
magick color. So, if you are meeting your lover,
or just want to exude a special attraction,
look up the day and wear something that
matches the corresponding shade.

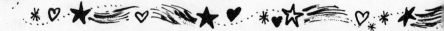

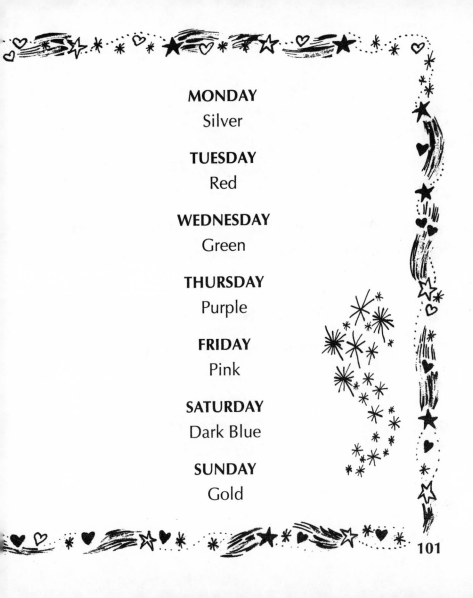

MONDAY
Silver

TUESDAY
Red

WEDNESDAY
Green

THURSDAY
Purple

FRIDAY
Pink

SATURDAY
Dark Blue

SUNDAY
Gold

Bye Bye Baby

What's a Love Goddess to do when Mr Right turns out to be Mr Wrong? To reverse a love spell or gently dissolve a relationship:

YOU WILL NEED TO GATHER:

A clean sheet of brown paper
A blue pen
A plate
A chopped onion
A chopped radish
Plastic wrap

Write their name on the piece of paper, and place it face-down on the plate. Cover with the chopped onion and radish, then cover with plastic, and leave in the fridge for seven days. On the eighth day, tip the paper, onion and radish into the plastic wrap to make a bundle and take it into a garden or a grove of trees. Sit and meditate for a few moments. Focus on relaxed and loving energy while you think about your ex-lover, and say:

'As I set you free, I do so wishing you kindness and friendship. May this spell help you on to your correct path, so you may find your true soul mate at last.'

Scatter the contents of the bundle over the garden or near the trees as you say: *'O Blessed Be.'*
(Don't forget to put the plastic wrap into a bin.)

Computer Cupid

What great magick the Internet is. Can you imagine what those ancient divas would have thought of surfing the Net and meeting potential partners through chat rooms? Powerful sorcery indeed! And a true Love Goddess never passes up an opportunity to weave her charms, even if it is with the aid of modern technology.

So, if you've got your eye on someone you've met on the Net, you can cast this attraction spell to give love a magickal boost. On the night of a full or growing moon, light some rose incense and then turn

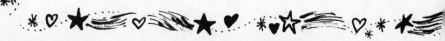

on your computer and open a new document which
you will call 'magick love spell'. Inside the
document, write down the name of your intended
lover and then type this incantation:

'Oh Mercury, spirit of communication and youth,
go swiftly with my request. Send my plea to the
Universal Goddess and aid me in my quest.
If love's spark is meant to be, when I speak his name
he will think of me, in the throes of passion he and
I will be. It shall be so, so mote it be.'

Say these words aloud to yourself each time you are
scheduled to meet him in the chat room.

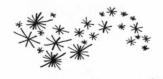

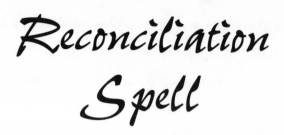

Reconciliation Spell

If you have had a lover's quarrel or wish to patch up a shaky relationship, you can cast this spell on a Wednesday evening around 7 o'clock.

YOU WILL NEED TO GATHER:

Cinnamon
Nutmeg
A glass bowl
A red cloth
A felt-tip pen
A red ribbon

Mix equal parts of cinnamon and nutmeg in a glass bowl as you recite this incantation:

'Gathering, gathering, come to the gathering, the powers to help me reconcile.'

Leave the mixture overnight, covered with a red cloth. In the morning, write your lover's name three times on the cloth with a felt-tip pen while you repeat the incantation again three times. Wrap the mixture up in the cloth, tie the ends with a red ribbon, and leave it in your bedroom drawer for as long as it takes.

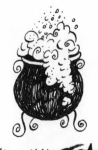

Hot Stuff

Do you wish to rekindle the flame of desire with your
husband or partner?

YOU WILL NEED TO GATHER:

*Hot spices (eg curry powder,
chili powder, paprika)*
A glass jar
A strand of your own hair
A strand of your lover's hair

One night, before your lover gets home, gather
together a few hot spices, like a teaspoon of curry,
a teaspoon of chili powder and a teaspoon of paprika,
and mix them together in a glass jar, and then put a
strand of your own hair and a strand of your lover's

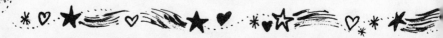

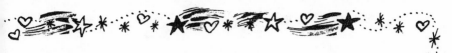

hair into the jar as well. Put on the lid tightly and shake it up as you repeat this incantation:

'As hot as fire is our desire, the love of life flows through our soul, when our bodies touch the flame ignites, this charge of lust will set things right.'

Place the jar of spices underneath your bed (where the hot and sexy magick will radiate upwards and through the entire bedroom), and then take a luxurious bath or shower and anoint your body with your best body lotions and perfumes. Take your time enjoying getting dressed in your sexiest clothes and underwear – really make a beautiful ceremony out of it. Then lie on your bed and feel your own Love Goddess energy surrounding you inside and out as you wait for your lover to arrive home. (The rest is up to your imagination!)

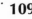

All that Glitters

Some of my most powerful spells include the energy of crystals and gems. Not only are these stones bright and alluring, but each one contains special and magickal attributes, helping you focus and strengthen enchantments for love and romance.

One of the easiest ways to choose a magickal crystal is to find your own birthstone through the help of the stars. Birthstone magick can be traced as far back as 4000 BC, to the spellcasters of Memphis, Egypt, who wore breastplates encrusted with special gems to protect and empower them with mystical energy.

Look up your star sign in the list opposite and find your matching love crystal.

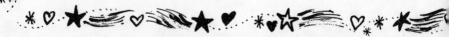

Wash your crystal in spring water mixed with a pinch of salt. Dry it well with a clean white cloth and keep this magick crystal in your pocket or on your desk.

AQUARIUS aquamarine
ARIES garnet
CANCER moonstone
CAPRICORN malachite
GEMINI agate
LEO amber
LIBRA lapis lazuli
PISCES amethyst
SAGITTARIUS topaz
SCORPIO tourmaline
TAURUS turquoise
VIRGO carnelian

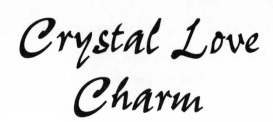

Crystal Love Charm

This Crystal Charm is for everyone who is ready to bring a special soul mate into their life.

YOU WILL NEED TO GATHER:

A rose-quartz crystal
Floral perfume
A red cloth

To help attract your perfect match, take the rose-quartz crystal and hold it close to your chest while you concentrate your thoughts on love and happiness. Feel your heart filling up with emotion as you say:

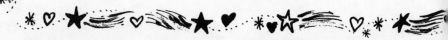

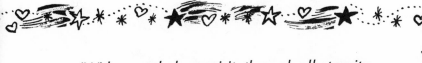

'With crystal clear spirit, through all eternity,
I open my mind and heart to receive true love.
So shall it be.'

Then spray the crystal with the floral perfume, wrap it in the red cloth, and keep it near your bed for one to three months.

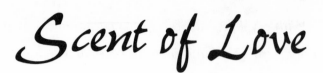

Scent of Love

Legend has it that Aphrodite invented one of the first fragrant love potions, which she carried around with her in a pouch spun from golden thread. The Roman goddess of love, Venus, is said to have given Helen of Troy a bottle of secret potion, which quickly turned her into the ultimate femme fatale.

Even the mere mortals of those ancient times were surrounded daily by the sexy scent of potent herbs and flowers (many of which we still use today). Love potions and perfumes were usually created with glorious mixtures of floral and herbal essences, and many included the essence of jasmine or even orange

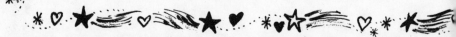

blossoms and pomegranates. The precious ingredients were then carefully mixed into oils, beeswax, or fine powders so as not to alter the magickal qualities of the pure floral and herbal essences. This is important, because the real power of a magickal perfume is retained not only in the aroma but also within the life force and vitality of the plants and flowers used.

Even in today's modern times, with the right ingredients and just a dash of enchantment, you can still stir up your own magick potion that will be guaranteed to unleash the love god (and goddess) in anyone!

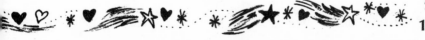

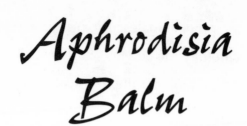

Aphrodisia Balm

YOU WILL NEED TO GATHER:

Rose essential oil
Neroli or orange essential oil
Ginger essential oil
One tablespoon of Vaseline (petroleum jelly)

Perfumes and scented body oils have been arousing lust and passion for centuries. This aphrodisia balm is a potent scent and quite expensive to make, but well worth it if you want to knock somebody's socks off.

On the night of a full or new moon, go to a private

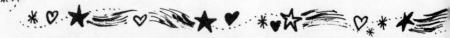

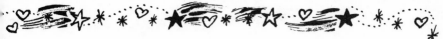

space in your home and put all your magick items on a flat surface. Undress and remain skyclad (witches' term for naked) during the spell. Put six drops of rose oil, six drops of neroli (or orange) and one drop of ginger into a clean, small glass jar. Mix in a tablespoon of petroleum jelly while you visualize the person you want to attract. Repeat this incantation:

> *'Magick of the ancient gods,*
> *Serve me well this lunar night*
> *And send me love on every breath*
> *Of this enchanted scent.'*

Dab a little of the balm on your wrists and behind your ears. Store the remaining balm in the jar (with the lid twisted on tightly) in the fridge to keep it fresh.

Perfumes of Eros

The ancient magicians knew that the aroma and vibrations from certain flowers and herbs help create an atmosphere of romance and seduction. Here are some of the most erotic and powerful aromas, along with their planetary correspondences. You can choose any one of these beautiful herbs and flowers, and either anoint a pink candle with the matching essential oil or simply sprinkle some dried or fresh flower/herb

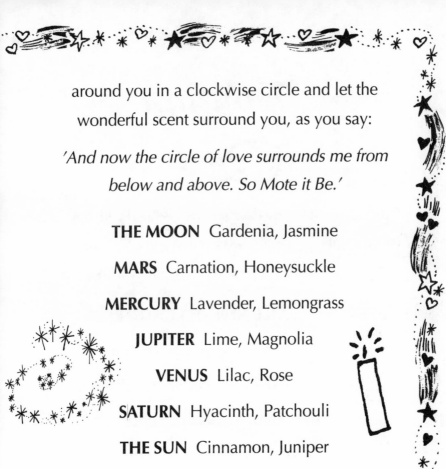

around you in a clockwise circle and let the
wonderful scent surround you, as you say:

*'And now the circle of love surrounds me from
below and above. So Mote it Be.'*

THE MOON Gardenia, Jasmine

MARS Carnation, Honeysuckle

MERCURY Lavender, Lemongrass

JUPITER Lime, Magnolia

VENUS Lilac, Rose

SATURN Hyacinth, Patchouli

THE SUN Cinnamon, Juniper

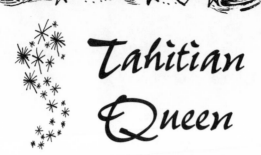

Tahitian Queen

If memories of balmy days and nights filled with the erotic scent of tropical flowers turns you on, this divine perfume will drive you and your guy crazy with desire.

YOU WILL NEED TO GATHER:

Quarter of a cup of coconut oil

6 drops of musk essence (or essential oil)

6 drops of gardenia essence

6 drops of frangipani essence

3 drops of sandalwood essence

Mix ingredients together well in a clean glass jar or container using a spoon or spatula. This beautiful scent is also a wonderful body and hair lotion, and you can smooth a generous amount over your entire body after bathing, or do as the sexy Tahitian girls do and comb some of the mixture through your hair like a fragrant hair gel. To add to the effect, wear a colorful sarong, place a red or white flower behind one ear, and get those hips of yours swinging to the jungle beat of love.

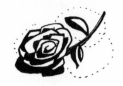

Moon Power

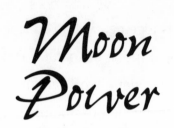

FULL MOON
For casting spells of love and high magick

NEW MOON
To begin a brand new relationship

WAXING OR GROWING MOON
To attract a soul mate or to strengthen a relationship

WANING OR DIMINISHING MOON
To end a relationship or to banish negative energy

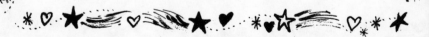

Deborah Gray

Australia's Good Witch was born into a long heritage of Celtic magick and mysticism. Initiated as a teenager into an Ancient Druid Circle, she has studied white witchcraft and alchemy for over twenty years, inheriting her knowledge of parapsychology and spellcasting from one of the world's few remaining Druid Masters.

As the author and co-author of the international bestsellers *Nice Girl's Book of Naughty Spells* and *How to Turn Your Ex-Boyfriend into a Toad,* Deborah is one of Australia's best known and respected writers. Her inspirational words of magick have been translated into four languages, exciting the imaginations of many thousands of people around the world.

In addition to her busy schedule as a metaphysical lecturer and writing for some of the world's leading publications, Deborah is passionately recreating the original perfumes and enchanted potions of ancient times, and has recently released her own Goddess of Love Potion.

For information on Deborah's catalogue or potions, please write to:
PO Box 229, Woollahra, NSW 2025 Australia
website: www.deborahgraymagic.com
e-mail: info@deborahgray.com